I0434398

Bible Diet, an Apple a Day

J.Z. Parker

Bible Diet, An Apple a Day

J. Z. Parker, Copyright C 2015

ALL RIGHTS RESERVED

The author is hereby established as the sole holder of the copyright.

Bible Diet, An Apple a Day

Table of Contents

Bible Diet, An Apple a Day

About the Author

J. Parker believes that each choice you make regarding your food lifestyle acts as either a deposit into or withdrawal from your "health banking" account. You can choose to make mostly savings deposits or check withdrawals. The balance of that account determines your energy, vitality, risk of disease, longevity, and ultimately the quality of your life.

J. Parker has worked in big food companies creating concepts. J.Z. is also a pseudonym. J. Parker, fondly referred to as J.P., writes to inspire a healthy relationship with food and exercise, along with practical tips to incorporate healthy living.

Bible Diet, An Apple a Day

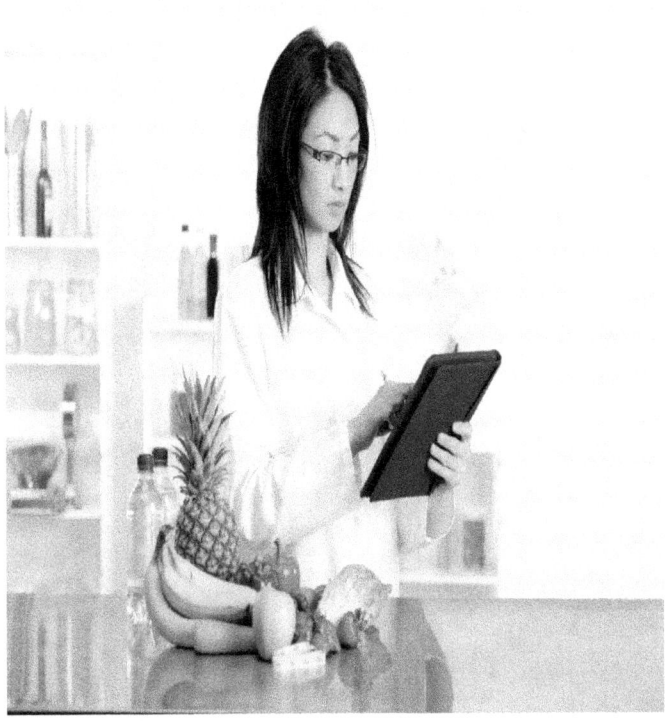

Bible Diet, An Apple a Day

Preface

There are 7.1 million deaths worldwide resulting from heart disease. That is greater than the population of some countries.

A few years back 7.9 million deaths were due to cancer.

In a few years it is estimated that cancer will claim 11million lives per year.

In the year 2031, 336 million people worldwide will be diabetic.

At the moment, 2/3 of Americans over the age of 20 are obese. In

UK, the government is considering declaring obesity as a disability. The above statistics are very scary yet intriguing. It has aroused my curiosity so much so that I became fascinated with the Biblical Methuselah.

There is a dynamic interplay in the story of Methuselah that has intrigued me recently. He chose, prepared, and consumed his foods like Adam--and like Adam he lived long, even longer than Adam.

Methuselah's age as recorded in the Bible has become the stuff of trivia, and debate. Have you ever wondered *why* he was the one who lived the longest? Like Adam, he lived a very long life.

If you really think about it, Methuselah's name is significant. It was so significant and meaningful because it translated to "When he dies, it will be sent." The *it,* was a euphemism for the big flood. It meant that Noah wasn't the only one to get the revelation concerning the destiny of the world. His great-grandfather Enoch was first to know.

Methuselah lived a total of 969 years, and then he died. Methuselah is the eldest son of Enoch recorded in the Bible (Genesis 5:21 KJV), the grandfather of Noah. But have you ever wondered why?

When Moses recorded the genealogy of Adam, the name

that commonly stands out in that list is Methuselah. Methuselah is the oldest person recorded in Scripture, and his name is often used today when referring to someone very old.

But was Methuselah a real human who lived? Some have come on the side of no. They opine that since he is not real, he could not be the oldest either. This is their theory. Methuselah was not the oldest man who ever lived, but he is the oldest man according to the Bible. Historians and anthropologists do not accept the biblical account of Methuselah's long life as literally true.

Whether historians and anthropologists agree or disagree for lack of evidence must not worry you. Evidence suggests that stories being peddled as ancient history cannot hold as true any longer today. Some of the stories have been found to be absolute fabrications or guesswork, as evidenced in many new archaeological findings. For one thing, there is a missing link in man's evolution history to the present-day man.

This missing link is between Neanderthals and Homo sapiens. Although the missing link has been there and explained in the Enuma Elish, the Bible too has a narration that man was created and/or re-engineered.

Good luck convincing any scientist to take a look at the information contained in those two mentioned sources: the Bible and Enuma Elish. Even when they look at other things that are non-spiritual, scientists most often will discard any theory unless it was Western-tested and approved.

What is still ironic and symptomatic of the conservative academic climate is that discoveries, theories, and evidence vigorously denied by the experts then can be accepted later, after it has been approved without a shadow of a doubt as a scientific truth. This was the same latter-day scientific truth which was regarded as a ridiculous proposition earlier.

This, therefore, is a permanent reminder of the intellectual apathy that reigned at earlier times. Such apathy still pervades the scientific cult society today, especially when it comes to matters rooted in the Bible. Sometimes, people in control never learn from the errors of our past.

Putting aside all of the environmental factors of a pre-flood world (where lifetimes lasted a lot longer than they do today), I'm convinced the answer has more to do with senescence: a state of unnoticed aging, a quality existing in Adam and

Eve's DNA before the Genesis 6:3 decision of God.

So why did God give Methuselah and a few others this quality to live for a lot many years—longer than anyone else in human history? What helped our progenitors live longer? Is it just senescence, or senescence enhanced by the food they ate? Was their DNA better than ours? There is research aimed at answering these and other questions. I was shocked at what I found, which has radically changed the way I choose and prepare my foods. I hope this book helps you too.

Bible Diet, An Apple a Day

Bible Diet, An Apple a Day

Chapter 1 Introduction: Methuselah's Long Life

If the biblical narratives were not heavy on food portions and ratios, we can learn that from the Maasai. Ratios mean how much of the categories of protein, fat, fruits, and carbohydrates we can eat. The Maasai tribe seems to have found a good balance. The Maasai are a very special people who live primarily from farming and livestock activities in Kenya and Tanzania.

My biology professor told me about their diets. My professor who is from the West and was then teaching at City University of New York (Lehman College) told a story of how he could not wait to visit his friends in East Africa. The Maasai, have mystified my researcher professor for years.

He spends eight weeks every year with them. He eats, showers, sleeps, and dresses like them while on the vacation. Whiteman dressed like a Maasai would be a sight to behold. My professor admitted to the class that he had yet to suffer any of his parents' illnesses, whereas all of his family siblings did.

To a large extent, the Maasai live on the milk from their cattle. This means that their diet is as full of fats as the diet of people living in the West. However, unlike Westerners, the Maasai do not have many problems related to lifestyle diseases. The Maasai eat greens on daily basis. Fruits direct from special trees are daily occurrences and happen on a whim. There is no encouragement needed to eat plenty of vegetables. Even the fattest Maasai are healthy.

The Maasai are nomads, so part of their daily routine entails walking--lots of it. Just walking. It is not even power walking-- just slow, regular strides. A study of the people found that on average, the Maasai walk/move

75 percent more than in the West where the activity level is about 44 kJ/kg/d, while for Maasai women the figure is 75 kJ/kg/d and for Maasai men it is 78 kJ/kg/d. The scientists registered activities of the walk-in kilojoules per kilo of body weight per day (kJ/kg/d).

Investigators in this new study have suggested that one of the reasons that the Maasai have lower rates of heart disease, despite a high-fat diet, is the amount of low-level aerobic activity they do on a daily basis. In doing their daily work of walking with the cattle they move around a lot at a slow pace. Just by walking, something most of us do not do any longer, they burn an astonishing 2500 calories a day in excess of their basal metabolic rate. The Maasai are not known to consume many carbohydrates—their carbohydrate intake is in quantities far less than we eat in the West.

The fact that they have a fairly low carbohydrate intake simply reaffirms that most of their energy demands come from the high amount of animal fat in their diets. At low level of aerobic activity, high carbohydrate intake is simply not necessary.

We have been taught to accept that a high-fat diet is bad for you, but you can see that the Maasai are not dieting like the West, which is high fat, high carbohydrates, and high protein, sometimes lacking fruits and vegetables.

The Maasai are capable of producing enough glycogen from the same high-fat, low-carb, and moderate- protein diet to fuel those long or short flashes whenever the need arises.

Our takeaway from the Maasai must be this: you can still eat high fat and be healthy by walking the fat away. A high-fat diet does not necessarily increase heart disease or death unless you accompany it with high carbohydrates, and thus, insulin.

 If you eat lots of fat, then reduce carbohydrate intake--*or* eat high carbohydrate and reduce your fat intake. This is simple enough.

You must take into consideration that even the earth moves. Can you imagine if the earth were still? You would have no seasons, no mornings, no afternoons, no nights. If the earth can move, so can you. Live well live long.

Chapter 2   Adam and Eve Had Super DNA

In some countries, the citizens are so slender that the few chubby ones are as a matter of culture viewed as "rich." In other countries, the overweight rate is so high that the few slender ones view obesity with overindulgence. Eating smart is the only way to better health.

It all boils down to proper nutrition. One book, the Bible, is the first to deal with nutrition and what and how to eat. One would then think that countries whose population is predominantly

Christian would logically have for its citizenry very healthy individuals: neither skinny nor fat, neither starving nor overweight. The question then follows: Are such countries following the biblical advice on diet? You could answer according to your convictions a yes or no, and make your call from there.

An observation made by a group of immigrants living in countries in the Western hemisphere in the USA is one worthy of study: Some of them who were struggling with their weight suddenly lost the weight on a four-week vacation to their homelands. One would ordinarily continue to wonder and ponder about the sudden weight-loss results until one learns the differences between the foods and how they were grown, packaged, and cooked. According to these now Dominican-Americans, Kenyan-Americans, Jamaican-Americans, Lithuanian Americans, and South African Americans, neither the eating habits nor the exercise habits changed.

However, they ate foods recommended in the Bible that their home countries had been eating for so long. They ate no hormones, no fertilizer, no re-engineered, and or/no modified foods. Many white, Americans especially those on the chubby side, who sought vacation in Kenya and neighboring countries returned to New York with stories of weight loss--an incentive to go back to Kenya, Tanzania and the neighboring countries' animal game reserves year after year. They were yearning to see the developments in the animals, but they also yearned for the enhanced weight loss they would experience again. To them, it was more than an experience. It was an expectation. Africa became a Mecca for unspoken weight loss experiences: a get-well destination.

We all hear, read, and see on TV, and in newspapers and magazines, what incredible things scientists are doing with and to DNA. Man has gotten to a level where we have come to understand DNA much better than we did many years ago. Man, it seems, is on geometric lane speeding to understand more about DNA.

With all the understanding of DNA, man has not even understood what 95% of the remaining chain of DNA does. It will take a very long time for scientists to fully come to grasp with all sections of the DNA.

But with the little of what man knows, we have started tinkering with DNA. Man is tinkering with DNA with intent to modify. Whether this is morally cool or not is not the premise of this book. Man also believes that chromosome rearrangements can play a role in whatever goal man chooses to pursue with regard to human re-engineering.

Now that we know that whatever you are has been coded in your DNA; now that we know that the color of your eyes has been coded in your DNA; now that we know that your ability to resist certain diseases has been encoded in your DNA, can we modify those characteristics? The answer is a resounding yes.

And yes, science is already employing these findings in our various life endeavors. As you read this and other narratives in the Bible or books like it, you need to understand what you read, for the words contained those books, if decoded correctly, are truths in plain view.

We read in the Genesis 3: [22]"And the LORD God said, Behold, the man is become as one of us, to know good and evil: and now, lest he put forth his hand, and take also of the tree of life, and eat, and live forever." He knew. He knew what man is capable of. He knew man's DNA, for we are part God. They re-engineered man. They knew.

Gen 6:3 "And the LORD said, My spirit shall not always strive with man, for that he also *is* flesh: yet his days shall be an hundred and twenty years."

And Gods Altered Man's DNA: Genesis 6:3.

This was a divine decree. And when God decrees it, so it shall be. Let us not jump ahead of ourselves. This verse meant and still means exactly what was decreed: the change in DNA. If we read what happened before this decree, you must have drawn a conclusion as to why God reached such a decision.

What your conclusion would be, depends strongly on whether you believe in the super intelligent beings that our ancestors have come to call gods. The gods pegged the human lifespan at 120 years +- a few years. Actually, it is mostly a minus. Up to minus (-) 119 years in some instances.

One thing I am sure of is that the decision to exterminate man from the face of the earth has nothing to do with man's lifespan. Man's lifespan of 120 years had been decreed by the gods before the decree to wipe man and beast off the face of the earth. This distinction must be made now because I do not subscribe to the analysis of pre-flood and after-flood lifespans.

One has nothing to do with the other. That only one family survived the flood in itself is a story for another day.

The Bible writers must come up with a narrative for why man's lifespan was shortened. The Bible also had to come up with excuse for the great deluge. The Bible had excuse for God's action in throwing Adam and Eve out of the garden. There were excuses or narratives.

The fascinating and interesting part is that it has always been same reason: SIN. Accordingly, man is full of sin. Always sinful. Man was so sinful that God decided to wipe His creation off of this earth.

Now, man must live only 120 years. Since then man's lifespan has been on the decline--or is it? Take a look at the table below. You may have observed that lifespans seem to decrease from Adam's era to Moses' era. There has been a steady decline from 930/950/969 to 120 or less.

Table of lifespan: Adam to Mosaic period

#	Name	Fathered a child at Age	Lifespan	Notes:
1	Adam	130	930	
2	Seth	105	912	
3	Enosh	90	905	
4	Kenan	70	910	
5	Mahalalel	65	895	
6	Jared	162	962	
7	Enoch	65	365 *	No death record
8	Methuselah	187	969	
9	Lamech	182	777	
10	Noah	500	950	
11	Shem	100	600	
12	Arphaxad	35	438	
13	Shelah	30	433	

14	Eber	34	464	
15	Peleg	30	239	
16	Reu	32	239	
17	Serug	30	230	
18	Nahor	29	148	
19	Terah	70	205	
20	Abram	100	175	
21	Moses		120	
22	Joshua		110	

- This author does not believe that Enoch died at age 365. He lived longer.

Does this decline in longevity suggest that the curse contained in the decree for a shorter lifespan been fulfilled? Not quite. If it proves anything, it proves the telomere theory, where we learned that when a cell divides, all of the DNA cannot be copied exactly and so a little gets cut off.

There is no total replication. Can this explain the reason to therefore say that Adam is more original to the initial DNA than present-day man? According to the Bible, Adam and Eve were created in God's image and likeness. They were highly resistant to disease and illness.

Their descendants would have inherited these advantages, albeit to lesser degrees. Over time, as a result of gene manipulation, the human genetic code became increasingly corrupted, and successive descendants lost their strong immune system and became more and more susceptible to disease and thus death. This would also have resulted in drastically reduced lifespans.

If one reads and understands the Bible well enough, it appears that non-senescence—not aging—was the original state of our progenitors. As if to support that understanding, there are some abnormal human cells today that do not age. These cells, sometimes called "immortal cells," presented a major headache to biologists interested in senescence, until it became clear that such cells were abnormal.

Today, some lines of cancer cells can be sustained in continuous culture through seemingly endless doubling. If scientists can determine how such abnormal cells survive, they may gain an insight into the process of cell aging.

Now that we are beginning to understand DNA, we can determine Adam's DNA; by understanding Adam's DNA, and how it relates to us, we can make some significant progress in understanding who we really are and how we found ourselves living shorter lives than our progenitors.

This means that he necessarily had all of the human genetic variations in his DNA. Like the Bible tells us, everyone, including Eve, came from Adam's DNA. Like we were also told by the Bible, every human being has two sets of genes: one from the father and the other from the mother. This could be an area that scientists could look into.

Now, how would the gods implement the decree? Was it difficult? Did it take a long span to implement? How did the gods implement it?

If you are science-inclined, you would have already guessed what the gods did. But scientists would not guess all. If you are the indoctrinated religious one, you may have been reading how the gods did it. You may however not think critically enough for the bulb to light up in your head.

All that the gods needed to do was tweak the area of the DNA that carried the information on how fast or slow the human body can age. They tweak it to where humans can survive up to 120 years and no more.

Another method the gods employed or could have employed is the use of diseases, such as **mitochondrial disease**. Mitochondrial disease is a group of disorders caused by dysfunctional mitochondria. Mitochondrial disease is caused by mutations in the mitochondrial DNA that affect mitochondrial function, thus weakening the immune system. Immune deficiencies may be temporary or permanent.

Temporary immune deficiency can be caused by a variety of sources that weaken the immune system. Common infections, including influenza and mononucleosis, can suppress the immune system. Primary immune deficiency diseases (PIDDs) are inherited genetic disorders and tend to cause chronic susceptibility to infection. There are over 150 PIDDs, and almost all are considered rare. They may result from altered immune signaling molecules or the complete absence of mature immune cells.

Some would say God would not do such things--so you might think. The gods have been and are still doing it today. Let us read evidence that confirms God's use of disease to achieve his goal. In Exodus, Pharaoh refused to let the Hebrew people go. Then plagues were rained on

Egypt. The ten plagues were thus narrated as a divine demonstration of Yahweh's powers and pleasure designed to persuade Pharaoh to let His people go.

One of the plagues was narrated in Exodus 9:3. "Behold, the hand of the LORD is upon thy cattle which is in the field, upon the horses, upon the asses, upon the camels, upon the oxen, and upon the sheep: there shall be a very grievous murrain." Another was when the livestock and man were diseased: Exodus 9:8-9. "And the LORD said unto Moses and unto Aaron, Take to you handfuls of ashes of the furnace, and let Moses sprinkle it toward the heaven in the sight of Pharaoh."

"And it shall become small dust in all the land of Egypt, and shall be a boil breaking forth with blains upon man, and upon beast, throughout all the land of Egypt." And if the diseases were not enough, the gods did the killing themselves. Here, read for yourself. 11:4-5: "And Moses said, thus saith the LORD, About midnight will I go out into the midst of Egypt:

"And all the firstborn in the land of Egypt shall die, from the first born of Pharaoh that sitteth upon his throne, even unto the firstborn of the maidservant that is behind the mill; and all the firstborn of the female servant who is behind the hand mill, and all the firstborn of the animals." Did they succeed? Let us see by cross-checking people from different eras. We will check the date of birth and how long they existed on earth:

#	Name	Born	died	Age
1	Abram			175
2	Moses			120
3	Joshua			110
4	George Washington	1732	1799	67
5	Galileo	1564	1642	77
6	Abraham Lincoln	1809	1865	56
7	Napoleon Bonaparte	1769	1821	51
8	James Madison	1751	1836	85
9	Ronald Reagan	1911	2004	93
10	Anwar Sadat	1918	1981	62

11	Obafemi Awolowo	1909	1987	78
12	Nelson Mandela	1918	2013	95
13	Nnamdi Azikiwe	1904	1996	91
14	Gabriel G. Marquez	1927	2014	87
15	Celia Cruz	1925	2003	77
16	Oscar de la Renta	1932	2014	82
17	Rafael Leonida Trujillo	1891	1961	69
18	Pope John Paul II	1920	2005	84
19	Elizabeth Taylor	1932	2011	79
20	Michael Jackson	1958	2009	50
21	Jeanne Calment	1875	1997	122*

- The maximum number of years an individual can live was set by God at 120. For humans, the current accepted maximum lifespan is 122 years achieved by Jeane

Clament of France. There are, however, claims to longer lives, but none have been acceptably documented.

Lifespan is different from life expectancy, which the average number of years a person can expect to live. Closing the gap between life expectancy and lifespan can be done through healthier living, less exposure to toxins, and also the prevention of chronic illnesses.

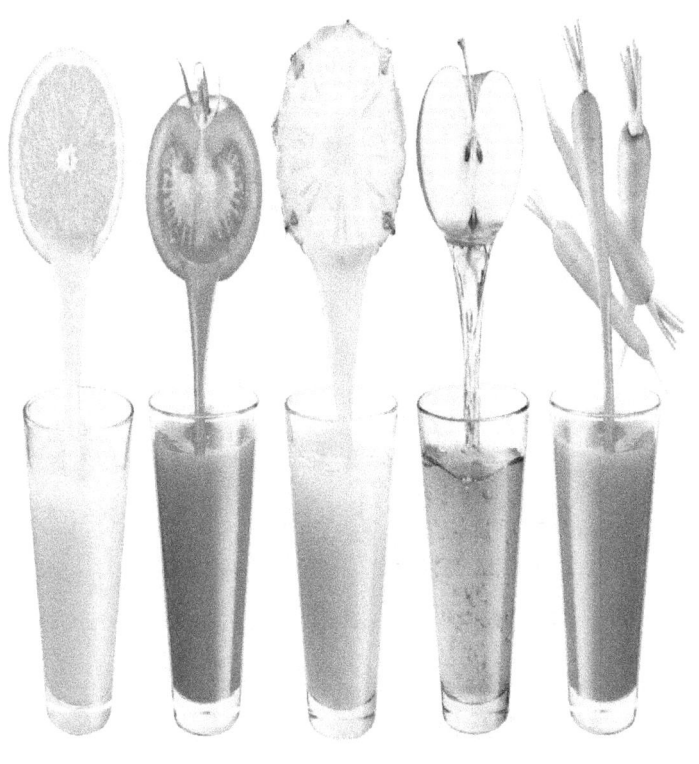

Chapter 3
The Telomere Theory

Let us check to see the effects of diet on aging. One theory in the theories of aging is the telomere theory. Telomeres are bits of DNA at the ends of chromosomes that shorten with cellular aging. Telomere length has been used as a marker for biological aging, chronic disease risk, and premature mortality.

Telomeres are sections of DNA at the ends of our chromosomes that protect the rest of the DNA each time a cell divides. When a cell divides, all of the DNA cannot be copied and so a little gets cut off. There is no total replication. Can this explain the reason that Adam is more original than, say, Cain and Abel?

Researchers have shown that older people have shorter telomeres. Eventually, the cells with shorter telomeres can no longer divide, and over time tissue damage and the dreaded "signs of aging" sets in. Cells can replicate approximately fifty times before the telomeres are too short.

It is however noteworthy to state here that cancer cells show a behavior that normal cells do not. Cancer cells do not die. They switch on an enzyme called telomerase, which adds to the telomeres when cells divide. There are some cells in our bodies that can also do this for example stem cells and sperm cells because they need to replicate more than fifty times in our lifetime.

We now know that our diet would affect this process. There are several studies that support this idea. Research finds that diabetics have short telomeres. In the journal *Diabetes Care* published by the American Diabetes Association, researchers discovered that the **telomeres of**

diabetics were significantly shorter than those without the disease.

Short telomeres for diabetics should not surprise us, but another study published in the journal *Atherosclerosis* found that even people who are *pre-diabetic* have shortened telomeres. They found that short telomeres trigger the *first sign of high blood sugar*.

It has been documented in a few studies that people who ate more vegetables and fruits had longer telomeres. Further analysis in some studies found a protective effect for a higher intake of vegetables only among overweight or obese women. We know that fruits and vegetables are rich in antioxidants, which help protect telomeres, extending the period for which they remain longer.

The takeaway from this theory: The length of telomeres within white blood cells is associated with human lifespan. Short telomeres are now associated with the development of chronic diseases of aging, including heart disease, diabetes, and some types of cancer.

Can we then draw the conclusion that diet helped the health of our forefathers? Can we also conclude that they lived a little longer then? We can answer yes. But can we

conclude that their longer life
was wholly due to diet? NO!

Would you then be surprised if I
said that you were fed from
birth to die rather than to live
longer, these days?

Bible Diet, An Apple a Day

Chapter 4 Adam and Eve Café

Let us fast-forward a couple of decades into the future. Our power to hack into life's software code (DNA) has advanced so rapidly that high school scholars can perform splicing experiments.

The rapid acceleration in biotech is due in no small part to the fact that we've harnessed bioscience into economic venture, thereby earning huge profits. It has become a way of thinking these days that the market is the main arbiter for deciding which biotechnologies enter the market.

Thus, if discoveries are made for immortality or longevity, Wall Street--including people of average savings--will dive into this market with their clothes on. It is not as if we have not modified other living things and are earning profits therefrom, such as with genetically altered foods. It's one thing to take a bioengineered drug. You know what you're getting and why.

Science and scientists seem to expect us to live for centuries and they are working toward it. In laboratories all over the world, scientists remove genes from experimental mice and rats and observe to see what happens. In gene splicing, they add genes to these same rodents and observe the results.

Today, not only is longevity theoretically possible, it is a scientifically achievable goal that can be attained in no time to benefit those of us alive today.

But our forefathers lived longer than we do. Why did they live longer?

If one were to base our conclusions as to why they lived longer on the sciences, we might arrive at wrong and misleading conclusions. This is so because while this author employs science concepts, man's science has yet to catch up with the gods. Man has made giant strides in the sciences, but there is more to learn. We are not like the gods yet. And even at that, most of our scientists scoffs at the mention of a Bible, thinking that the Bible has nothing to offer in the area of science, specifically in area of biology. But that is far from the truth.

    a. Adam lived side-by-side with the gods. Adam saw the gods. Adam spoke with the gods. Most importantly, Adam learned from the gods. The gods walked like man does and Adam described that in Genesis 3:8-12. So, for the length of time Adam lived, there was the period he was young and a period he grew old. Like all healthy humans, he learned as he grew and he learned from the gods. Where he failed in the rules and regulations, he was either corrected and or punished. One example of what he learned from the gods was diet. This was well documented in the book of Genesis more than once. Genesis 1:29-30:

"[29]And God said, Behold, I have given you every herb bearing seed, which *is* upon the face of all the earth, and every tree, in the which *is* the fruit of a tree yielding seed; to you it shall be for meat.

"[30] And to every beast of the earth, and to every fowl of the air, and to   everything that creeps upon the earth, wherein *there is* life, *I have given* every green herb for meat: and it was so.

> "31 And God saw everything that he had made, and, behold, *it was* very good.

Something was missing in Adam's diet. Meat and fish. Bloody stuff. Adam's diet was purely vegetarian. Did you know this earlier? In fact, in those early days, even the beasts of the earth were strictly on vegetarian diet. Adam and Eve's Café/restaurant is exactly the garden.

There were no deep fryers. Their French fries were an apple or mango. They had no high-calorie foods and just the attempt to go to the restaurant/café was enough exercise. No trainer had to tell Adam and Eve to work out, as they usually would get plenty of exercise with their standard daily duties no matter how many veggies they consumed.

Adam and his woman had no refrigeration, so their food was obtained from the source--very fresh, no preservatives added. Adam's physical Ed trainer was Yahweh Himself. He had an original design for Adam and Eve. Their daily routine was organized thus:

1. They had to walk a few miles to go to the fruit café.
2. There were no short cuts to the food. Thus there was a daily exercise.
3. The diet and exercise were inseparable.

4. They eat as much as they wanted, except the fruits belonging to "the tree of knowledge."

5. We do not know whether Adam and Eve were given supplements of the gods. Do not discount this, for as we know, Adam and Eve had direct contact and God's supervision.

What Adam and Eve's diet could look like today, and where they would walk to get their food:

a. Veggie markets--this is not even available in all locales today

b. Trees of various types with fruits

c. Salads

    d. Palm nuts, melons, melon seeds, vegetable leaves.
    e. Fish markets
    f. Fats and carbs will be at the bottom: yams, plantains, beans, rice, cocoyam etc.

Now most nutritionists today would talk about and highlight the nutritional values of fruits and thus the need to eat more of them. We now know that fruits are high in natural carbohydrates and sugar, especially fructose, as opposed to sucrose found in refined sugar.

They are a very good source of many varieties of vitamins, minerals, and of course fiber. We also understand now that another second food variety would be raw nuts of all kinds: these include almonds, walnuts, pecans, and pistachio nuts. Nuts in general contain monounsaturated fat and polyunsaturated fats.

They are a good source of protein and vitamins, particularly vitamin E. They also are filled with minerals such magnesium, phosphorus, iron, and fiber.

So far all evidence points to a vegetarian diet as a layman would describe it. Some call it a vegan diet. A vegan diet is one that is prepared without animal components. What must be taken from the Bible's description of all the foods God allowed our early ancestors is that they came with no animal fats. However, things were about to change. Soon after the floods, Noah killed some animals and offered burnt offerings on the altar and the Lord smelled a soothing aroma. So began the consumption of meat.

And soon, God confirmed or gave permission to human beings to eat flesh. God told Noah and his sons, "Every moving thing that lives shall be food for you. I have given you all things, even as the green herbs." (Genesis 9:3)

So after the Flood, God definitely cements the permission to humans to eat "every moving thing that lives." And there was no more record of humans living up to 900 years and beyond like

Adam or Methuselah. But was the permission to eat meat the cause of the reduction in longer life? That is the question, and we must find out.

Chapter 5
Genetically Modified
Foods (GMO)

It is worth mentioning that the best scientists--the gods--saw no need for GMOs, though one could argue that there weren't so many mouths to feed then. Adam and Eve, Noah and his family, and Methuselah did not eat modified foods.

You cannot tell a genetically modified apple--neither can I. An average Joe goes to the supermarket and buys whatever apples and oranges are displayed. We choose whatever chicken is available. Where available, organic is not for the average Joe because it is priced out of reach. Do you think that it would be fair to ask farmers/retailers to identify how they grew their products? Is it fair to the farmers?

Organic product farmers proudly announce to everyone and at every opportunity that their product is organic. They must know what was divinely ordained.

Have you heard of the maxim "You reap what you sow?" Or GIGO, the information technology acronym for "Garbage in, garbage out"? While several parties defend the benefits and use of technology to create an abundance of food, it follows that little is being done to inform the end consumer of long-term effects in consuming fertilizer-packed and genetically tampered-with apples and oranges.

It is estimated that as many as 60 to 70 percent of all foods sold in US grocery stores and supermarkets may contain some genetically modified foods. Soybeans and corn, common ingredients in a number of processed foods, are the most common genetically modified plants in the United States agricultural sector. As if to add to consumers' confusion, the Food and Drug Administration considers genetically modified foods equivalent to naturally grown (organic) foods.

Whether we are adversely affected by GMOs is not why they are mentioned in this book. Genetically modified foods are mentioned to serve as a reminder to you that those who came before us--namely Adam, Seth, Enosh, Enoch, and Methuselah-- did not eat GMOs.

So, what exactly is genetically modified food? It is the introduction of or inserting of different genes not normally found in a given food or plant. Inserting genes not normally found in a certain food or plant results in a genetically modified food. When this is done, it could result to a different kind of food. This is genetically modified, and therefore, tampering.

The gods warned against such foods in Genesis 7:14 where emphasis is laid on classification: kind after their kind.

Chapter 6   120-Year Lifespan

There are a few peoples who live well into a hundred years and above, including the Ikarians in Greece, the Maasai in Tanzania/Kenya, the Fulanis of West Africa, and women of the Island of Okinawa. On Costa Rica's Nicoya Peninsula, there exists a small population of approximately100, 000 mestizos with a lower-than-normal rate of middle-aged mortality; and finally and probably not the last, there are the members of the Seventh Day Adventist Church in

Loma Linda, California, USA where it has been observed that the population of these Seventh-Day Adventists adherents has a life expectancy that exceeds the American average by about a decade.

There is a connection of truth among these people. They eat divinely recommended foods. They do so knowingly and unknowingly. The strongest link among them is their longevity enhanced by their diet. All the diets are summarized in the Seventh-Day Adventists' type of diet-- the healthful plant-based diet. This Seventh-Day Adventists' diet has been associated with an extra decade of life expectancy.

The diet of all these people has been linked to reduced rates of diabetes and heart disease, and thus increased longevity. Like this book, the Seventh-Day Adventists' diet is inspired by the Bible, specifically Genesis 1:29-30.

"²⁹And God said, Behold, I have given you every herb bearing seed, which *is* upon the face of all the earth, and every tree, in the which *is* the fruit of a tree yielding seed; to you it shall be for meat.

"³⁰ And to every beast of the earth, and to every fowl of the air, and to everything that creeps upon the earth, wherein *there is* life, *I have given* every green herb for meat: and it was so."

If it is green and fit for consumption, eat it and beat it.

The Adventists have been eating the way they do for decades. It does not hurt that Adventists mostly keep as friends other Adventists; thus there are no distractions from their way of life. No drinking. No smoking. No drugs.

Have you ever thought of following the diet in the Bible? We were told what foods to eat. When the Bible's hallowed screams on failed diets remain hidden, its truth on "good foods," backed by facts, seems always to assert itself for those who are able to find its recommendations. Again and again, research tends to arrive at a conclusion reached thousands of years ago by the Bible.

Do you know this diet? Being well-fed does not lead to healthy living. Some nations are overfed yet undernourished, while some seem to be underfed yet healthier. How and where do you find the middle ground to feed well and be well- nourished and healthy? We are still finding the answer to this question thousands of years after our progenitors— Adam, Eve, or Methuselah. We are still at the stage of experimentation where what was good for you yesterday is bad for you today. Tomorrow, such food could be good or bad, depending on who is producing and selling it.

We are still in the science of cholesterol. Cholesterol was bad for you yesterday and today; LDL is a bad cholesterol while HDL is a good cholesterol. LDL cholesterol is considered the bad cholesterol because it contributes to plaque buildup--a thick, hard deposit that can clog arteries and make them less flexible-- while HDL cholesterol is considered a good cholesterol since it enhances the removal of LDL cholesterol from the arteries.

Scientists believe HDL acts as a scavenger, carrying LDL cholesterol away from the arteries. It was a scientific leap in discoveries then. The abundance and make-up of your cholesterol partly depends on the foods you shove down your throat.

A journey into a bookstore, a library, or the worldwide web will leave you with the impression that avoiding most human diseases is a matter of properly choosing what goes inside your tummy. In both places (bookstore and internet) you will read about the benefits of foods with magical powers to prevent all kinds of diseases that ail man. Some claim that certain foods have such powerful protective nutrients, such as antioxidants and other derivatives. Sometimes, the readers are directed to pursue a diet that is simple and primitive, like those of some Chinese or Japanese peasants. Some have long dismissed such diets as fit only for the Paleolithic cave dwellers.

But cave dwellers or not, science is now bridging the gap of misunderstanding in our dietary needs. Adam and Eve and/or Methuselah could have been a myth, just like the way they fed themselves for sustenance could be described as nutritional folklore.

When I use the word "myth," I do not mean fable. I want it to mean oral histories passed to us by our fathers whose fathers passed same to them. The truth was and still is that Adam and others, though Paleolithic cave dwellers, were "divinely" instructed as to what to eat and not eat.

Though primitive as we describe their diets today, science is opening our eyes to foods that have nutrients that nourish and foods that destroy and incapacitate human well-being. Though they were Paleolithic cave dwellers, they never engaged in guessing as to which food was good like we do today. These days the scene is like this:

yesterday, we read that iron was good for you. Today, you read another source saying that too much iron is bad because the body cannot filter and dispose of excess iron.

Methuselah was 969. Nelson Mandela was 95.

Adam was 930. George Washington was 67.

Moses was 120. Michael Jackson was 50.

As you can observe, there was and still is a geometric decrease in lifespan from Adam to Genesis 6:3. The decreed 120 years was unmistakably explained in Genesis 6:3.

Chapter 7
Shorter and Shorter Lives

Lifespan is the maximum number of years an individual from a given species can live. For Homo sapiens, the current accepted maximum lifespan is 122 years. This is not made-up. It is real and achieved. This was achieved according to Guinness book of records by Jeane Clament of France.

There are some other claims to longer lives, but none of these have been properly documented and accepted. Lifespan is different from life expectancy, which is the average number of years a person can expect to live. But there is good news. The good news is that closing the gap between life expectancy and lifespan can be done through healthier eating and living, with less exposure to toxins and sicknesses.

Why were the lifespans of people living in biblical times so much longer than they are today? What has changed? Why did people in the Old Testament live for hundreds of years before the Flood? Our lifespans dropped dramatically after the Flood. Have you noticed? There is no debating that fact, science- or religion- wise. Why do people living today live much shorter lifespans than in the days of Adam and Methuselah?

 Why don't we eat like Adam? Is it such harder to eat like our progenitors?

I have had this question asked so many times and I had no answer. Then, I reread the book *Why Was Man Created?* I got an insight. I saw that the gods were scientists too, among other fields occupationally.

I got an insight that God Himself is a surgeon and biological engineer. Before you ask me how and why I knew that, let us read Genesis 2:21. By now, you must have come to the understanding that I take some evidence from the Bible. I do not think that the Bible narratives were the figment of the prophets' imaginations.

In the book of creation, Genesis 2:21, we read of how God performed a surgical operation on Adam and took a rib. To a non-understanding individual, God just took a rib. To a critical mind, God took a rib that contained DNA which He modified to create a woman.

Now, the word modify is very important here, especially when discussing how our foods are produced. This will be so because I want to avoid all the science and biological jargon which we may find difficult to understand. Another word that would be that important is DNA. The first few humans recorded in the Bible lived an exceedingly long time.

Adam lived to the age of 930 years, his son Seth lived to be 912, and then his son Lamech lived 777 years. Lamech's son Noah in turn lived to 950 years, his son Shem lived 600 years. As you can notice, there was an emerging pattern.
Progressively, each generation lived shorter and shorter lives. Adam was the first human created/re-engineered and must have been nearly perfect. Adam was the result of modification. Modified humans were more

perfect in health, size, and stature.

It follows that the first generations of humans lived such long lives because they were so close--nearer in DNA--to the man (Adam) that God created, and what God created seemed perfect from the beginning.

There was no clear-cut understanding, then or now, about whether man was created with intent to live forever. If anyone should be in the know, I should, because I researched that topic and wrote a book on it. In that book, a reason for the creation of man was surmised and documented. Now, from that, we know that man could not have been created to live forever.

He was created for a purpose, but he was not created to live forever. Let us see some evidence. Genesis 3: "¹⁹ In the sweat of thy face shalt thou eat bread, till thou return unto the ground; for out of it was thou taken: for dust thou *art*, and unto dust shalt thou return.

"²⁰ And Adam called his wife's name Eve; because she was the mother of all living.

"²¹ Unto Adam also and to his wife did the LORD God make coats of skins, and clothed them.

"²² And the LORD God said, Behold, the man is become as

one of us, to know good eat, and live forever:

"23 Therefore the LORD God sent him forth from the Garden of Eden, to till the ground from whence he was taken.

"24 So he drove out the man; and he placed at the east of the garden of Eden Cherubims, and a flaming sword which turned every way, to keep the way of the tree of life."

Reading the above verses tell us what we need to know about our mortality. It tells us that we will die at some point. To totally achieve this objective, the "tree of life," or the secret DNA codes, were hidden in a Cherubim.

If you have read my other books, you must know by now what a Cherubim is. If it tickles your fancy, you can call this DNA the "tree of life."

The tree of life was and still is simply the web of DNA codes. There was no tree. There was no angel as in cherubim and there was no flaming sword; however, there was something flaming in the blades that turned every way to keep intruders away. Even the helpers in the Garden of Eden could not get to the cherubim once the "tree of life" was placed in them.

When the tree of life was placed in the cherubim, it eliminated any chance that man could ever be immortal. We may wonder

whether it was the gods'
intention to modify man to
become immortal. That could be
so, for as read from the Bible
initially, Adam and Eve were
created.

Later, the Bible said Adam was
created without Eve. According
to the Bible, no companion could
be found for Adam. So God took
Adam's DNA, which He
modified to arrive at Eve. The
watchword is "modification."
Another word is "re-engineer."
The gods were tweaking man's
DNA.

They could therefore tweak how
many years we can live. This
must not come as a surprise; after
all, our present-day scientists are
tweaking the DNA of various

animals, including human. We can therefore see that man was initially made to live for a period of time with room for modification. That modification could have gone either way.

There would have been a chance for immortality or mortality. Out of anger, man was punished to a short life--considering how long those intelligent beings lived, man's life was about to take a turn for the worse. The chance for that modification to immortality was closed when Enki the scientist tweaked man to become as intelligent as the gods. He achieved that feat by tweaking the "tree of life." That tree of life has now been locked away. Read Genesis 3:22 above.

We can read the about many men (our forefathers) who lived a healthier and longer life than we do. Here are some of them as documented the Bible.

•So all the days of Seth were nine hundred and twelve years, and he died. (Gen. 5:8)
•So all the days of Enosh were nine hundred and five years, and he died. (Gen. 5:11)
• All the days of Kenan were nine hundred and ten years, and he died. (Gen. 5:14)
• All the days of Mahalalel were eight hundred and ninety-five years, and he died. (Gen. 5:17)
• The days of Jared were nine hundred and sixty-two years, and he died. (Gen. 5:20)
• The days of Methuselah were

nine hundred and sixty-nine
years, and he died. (Gen. 5:27)
•So all the days of Lamech were
seven hundred and seventy-seven
years, and he died. (Gen. 5:31)

Chapter 8
Negligible
Senescence

Is it then a mystery that people in early chapters of Genesis lived longer lives while 150,000 years later, we croak at 120? There are many theories put forward by biblical scholars.

The genealogy in Genesis 5 records the line of the godly descendants of Adam—the line that would eventually produce the Messiah. God possibly blessed this line with especially long life as a result of their godliness and obedience.

While some would want to pull wool over people's eyes, we know that we can draw any genealogical lines we intend to draw. For example, if the records were available, you the reader could draw your lines to Adam and Eve no matter your lineage.

So, this theory is a "divine" fluke. While this is a possible explanation, the Bible nowhere specifically limits the long lifespans to the individuals mentioned in Genesis Chapter 5.

In fact, other than Enoch, Genesis 5 does not identify any of the individuals as being especially godly. The record at the time simply evidenced a simple truth: they all lived several hundred years. It is therefore sensibly reasonable to look for the factors that made it so.

Several factors could have contributed to this. Though evidence is lacking, we can read a trend and thus make reasonable deductions. If you connect the dots, the answer is there in plain sight, staring at those who read the Bible. The gods simply tweaked that part of our DNA responsible for timing growth, the immune system, and death. They reset the human time clock.

Some have reasoned that because Genesis 1:6-7 mentions the water above the expanse, a mass of water that surrounded the earth that would have created a greenhouse effect and would have blocked much of the radiation that now hits the earth. This would have resulted in ideal living conditions. I do not buy this explanation.

Though I am not a scientist, evidence abounds that narrates the arrival of the gods. If such canopy of waters existed, one would only wonder how the gods passed through. If such waters exist, I wonder why it is not hampering NASA's flights to other planets.

To drive home this canopy of water in the sky theory, some point to Genesis 7:11 and proclaim that it indicates that at the time of the Flood, the water canopy was poured out on the earth, ending the ideal living conditions. And they ask you to compare the lifespans before the Flood (Genesis 5:1-32) with those after the flood (Genesis 11:10-32).

Immediately after the Flood, the ages decreased dramatically. What they fail to add is though ages decreased after the Flood, ages had been decreasing right from Adam. However, the most reasonable and logical explanation is that the gods tweaked man's DNA. The gods equally did not hide it, for immediately before the Flood, the gods decreed a 120-year lifespan for man.

One more consideration is that in the first few generations after creation, the human genetic code had developed few defects. Adam and Eve were created perfectly to age slowly or perhaps not age at all— something science refers to as senescence or non-senescence.

Senescence simply means growing into old age very slowly, while non-senescence is growing old so slowly that it is hardly noticed. There is an emerging area of aging research of long-lived animals with negligible senescence. Scientists have found that in many animals the aging process is so slow that it is either nonexistent or too slow to be measured reliably in the laboratory.

One scientist whose name comes up on this research is Caleb Finch of USC. "Negligible senescence" is what Caleb Finch nicknamed this slow-aging or non-aging process.

Thus the animals that exhibit negligible senescence don't have a finite lifespan like other animals. Now I know why the turtle appears in many moonlight tales as the wisest animal for its longevity.

From Caleb Finch's studies we now know that *"animals, that exhibit Negligible Senescence, don't have a finite lifespan like other animals. Which means they don't have a maximum age of life where they would die of old age.*

They also seem to resist the diseases of old age. They have a life expectancy, or live to an age to which they die of disease, predators, or starvation- but not old age. In this sense, these animals can be considered immortal. Perhaps just as interesting, these animals do not have a fixed body size (such as some lobsters, flounders, sturgeons, sharks, alligators. turtles, and whales) they simply increase in body size with time while showing no noticeable sign of aging."

You may be surprised that such information is out there. Though the study of long-lived animals is still new to aging research, more investigations and research must be conducted so as to enable a conclusive scientific evidence. Caleb Finch said, "I think we're pretty far away from finding the answers we are seeking. There are a lot of mechanisms that determine lifespan. No one is paramount. Even with such studies, I don't expect a quick and easy answer, potion, or elixir. I do know we can learn more about aging by studying animals with lifespans longer than humans."

Meanwhile, conducted researches show that whales can live over 200 years. An example is the bowhead whale, a baleen whale, perhaps the oldest mammal on the planet, which has been found to be over 210 years old.

Even zoos in various places have compiled longevity information. Alligators have been recorded to live up to eighty years of age, while we are not sure if death was due to senescence or environmental factors. It is widely expected that older alligators also do exist. Green sea turtles take up to fifty years to reach maturity in the wild. Scientists are still studying and documenting some other facts about green sea turtles' lifespan. It is believed that it will be much greater than previously thought.

A research study was done by the Alaska Fish and Game Department. The study provided data on some randomly sampled yellow eye rockfish, commercially caught off of the coast of Alaska. The study showed that about 16 percent of the fish were 50 years of age. Some were older than 100 years old.

That there are in existence animals with no fixed lifespan seems to indicate that *age genes* do not exist for them, or that aging is so slow for some animals it seems they do not age, unlike humans. What this means is simply that the cells of these animals never lose their vigor or their ability to reproduce. The cellular structure and its functions, the DNA and its chromosomes of these non-aging animals has become the research goals of scientists in the hopes to finding the "fountain of youth" for Homo sapiens.

It is as if the pronounced injunctions in Genesis 6:3 do not affect many other living things. That pronouncement is for man alone. Think about it. The trees live longer too, though they mostly die of diseases.

Another study by a German research group found that lobsters produce lots of telomerase and show very slow signs of aging during their long lives. Telomerase prevents the decay of telomeres, which caps the end of chromosomes.

As explained in an earlier chapter, human cells usually

divide about 75 times over a lifetime. Each time a cell divides, the telomeres erode, thereby making them shorter. When this happens, the cell can no longer divide, and eventually dies. This study therefore suggests that telomerase has some kind of anti-aging property that protects cells.

Good food and health help the telomerase stay longer for a longer period of time before it divides. It does not end there. There is yet another study that is bordering on immortality. The question is: Can science, through the study of animals whose cells divide more than 75x, find a way to trick our cells by introducing those other cells that disobey the number of times the cells must divide?

Another study by Dr. Daniel Martinez, Associate Professor of Biology and Coordinator of the Molecular Biology Program of Pomona University, seeks to understand the role of telomerase in protecting the somatic cells of the hydra, a type of metazoan. Martinez also touts the enzyme telomerase as one of the factors in the hydra's negligible senescence and possible immortality.

Meanwhile, I must emphasize that there is still very little information on this budding field of study. It will be fascinating to follow along with the research as it is made available by the scientific community to the public. You may have observed that these animals mentioned mostly live in water.

Chapter 9   Fasting as a Method for Dieting

If you are obese and struggling, it's never too late to start over. If you weren't happy with yesterday, try something different today. Don't stay stuck. You can always do better.

Though I have no scientific evidence that our progenitors fasted, one cannot rule out that they experienced periods of controlled starvation, otherwise known as fasting involuntarily.

Today, many Christians and other religious adherents engage in intermittent fasting, voluntarily. Some do a forty-day fast. Some do a thirty-day fast. Some do a periodic weekly fast, while some fast once a week. Jesus Christ Himself was known to partake in fasting. If Jesus did that, learn from it if you are a Christian.

We usually eat three square meals a day while also chowing down on snacks all day long. Instead of eating three square meals a day, an eating schedule that involves intermittent fasting can help fight not just obesity but other related diseases such as diabetes, heart disease, cancer, and Alzheimer's.

Consuming fewer calories and exercising more has been the usual advice we receive from nutritionists. Such advice highlights the benefits of such foods as vegetables, fruits, nuts, fiber, and fish, and the value of reducing or eliminating snacks.

However, mounting evidence reveals that another key aspect of diet--fasting--can also play a major role in health. Many research studies show that intermittent fasting could have benefits, but often, nutritionists hardly advise clients to follow the route of fasting as part of their dieting practice.

Fasting alone is more powerful in preventing and reversing some diseases like obesity and related diseases, thus eliminating such diseases and enhancing longevity more effectively than drugs.

There are many benefits to this practice. Engage in fasting because you will benefit and gain antiaging effects, you will have better attitude, better resistance to disease and better sleep--and most importantly, you gain a much-needed change in habits.

I will list the benefits of fasting I hope you incorporate this method of dieting into your weekly, monthly, or yearly plans as lots of evidence indicates that timed periods of fasting are a good thing. Fasting has been called the "miracle cure" because the list of physical conditions improved by fasting is long and varied. Cited most often are allergies, arthritis, digestive disorders of all kinds, skin conditions, cardiovascular disease, and asthma. Fasting will:

1. Rest the digestive system
2. Allow for cleansing and detoxification of the body
3. Create a break in eating patterns, while shining a spotlight on them
4. Promote greater mental clarity
5. Cleanse and heal "stuck" emotional patterns
6. Lead to a feeling of physical lightness, increasing your energy level
7. Promote an inner stillness, enhancing spiritual connection

8. Spiritually, when you fast, you see clearly

Fasting has become increasingly popular over the years, especially among health communities. Though some health practitioners are afraid to recommend eating less or fasting, due to the stigma of religion involved, intermittent fasting has lots of medical benefits when used sensibly.

Here are some more benefits in detail to help you incorporate fasting as part of your diet.

It is naturally obvious that fasting helps weight loss. Fasting may be a safe way to lose weight, as many studies have shown that intermittent fasting—fasting that is controlled within a set number of hours—allows the body to burn off fat cells more effectively than just regular dieting. Less is taken in; therefore there is less to burn. Intermittent fasting forces the body to use fat as primary source of energy instead of sugar.

Meanwhile, fasting helps balance your insulin sensitivity. Fasting has a positive effect on insulin sensitivity, allowing you to tolerate carbohydrates (sugar) better. It follows that after periods of fasting, insulin becomes more effective in telling cells to take up glucose from blood. That is not all. It helps speed up the metabolism.

Intermittent fasting is a recess kind of break for the digestive system, and this can energize your metabolism to burn off calories more efficiently. If your digestion is inefficient, it can affect your ability to metabolize food and burn fat. Intermittent fasts can regulate your digestion and promote healthy bowel function, thus improving your metabolic function.

Aging hates fasting because fasting enhances longevity. From earlier chapters you may have observed that to maintain good health, you eat less. Believe it or not, the less you eat the healthier and longer you will live.

Studies have shown how the lifespan of people in certain countries and cultures increased due to their diets/cultures, which may include fasting. One of the primary effects of ageing is a slower metabolism so the less you eat, the less burden on your digestive system. Fasting also improves hunger.

Fasting enables you to regulate the hormones in your body. When you are obese, you fail to receive correct signals as to when to stop eating. Your impulses misfire. Fasting therefore serves as your alarm. The more you fast, the more your body can regulate itself to release the appropriate hormones that enables you to experience what real hunger is.

When your hormones are working efficiently, you get full quicker too.

Fasting improves eating patterns. Fasting can be a helpful practice for those who suffer from eating disorders such as binge eating. If you are on a seven-day fast, it is very likely that you will break your fast, the same time every day, thus establishing a correct eating pattern whether or not you work and have other priorities.

Fasting will also improves brain functions. Fasting has shown to improve brain function, as it enhances the production of a protein called brain-derived neurotrophic factor (BDNF.) BDNF induces brain stem cells to convert into new neurons, thus triggering numerous other chemicals that promote neural health. BDNF also protects brain cells from changes associated with Alzheimer's and Parkinson's disease.

Here are two more benefits why you should do intermittent starving. It improves the immune system, regulates inflammatory conditions in the body, and starves off cancer cell formation.

Fasting contributes to self-enlightenment as it helps your connection to life through meditation, yoga, and other activities. With no food in the digestive system, this makes room for more energy in the body – the digestive process is one of the most energy-absorbing systems in the body.

Fasting for 8-12 hours period makes you wonder, realize, and empathize with those who starve over a long period of time all over the world. It makes you appreciative and grateful for life's little things.

Fasting prevents acne. This is because with the body temporarily freed from digestion, it focuses its regenerative energies on other systems. Not eating anything for just one day has shown to help the body clean up the toxins and regulate the functioning of other organs of the body like the liver, kidneys, and other parts.

Chapter 10
Conclusion

The apple is a gift. So are the many other fruits. The apple is gift that keeps giving. It is left to you to receive and keep receiving. An apple a day keeps the doctor away. How? I am used to hearing the mantra "An apple a day keeps the doctor away."

That mantra is of course better than "Take two aspirin and call me tomorrow morning." The apple is a very special fruit. It is so special that you would never hear an orange or a banana a day keeps the doctor away. This is so because apples have properties that are like no other fruit.

Though other fruits combined would give you benefits like an apple, how many people have the patience to sit and eat all those other fruits?

An apple combines many vitamins and benefits in one punch. That makes it easy for most people. When it is made simple, easy, and fast, people go for it in an attempt to take care of their health. What makes an apple so special?

Apples are rich in flavonoids, which help to prevent heart disease. Flavonoids are also shown to have antioxidant effects. Many flavonoids are known to have anti-oxidative activity, free-radical scavenging capacity, coronary heart disease prevention ability, and anticancer activity, while some flavonoids exhibit potential for anti-human immunodeficiency virus functions.

Apples also contain phenols, which helps to reduce bad cholesterol while increasing good cholesterol. Apples help prevent LDL cholesterol from turning into oxidized LDL, a very dangerous form of bad cholesterol. One study thinks a benefit comes from pectin, a powerful fiber that clings to cholesterol and sweeps it out of the body. This study recommended green apples.

A study has it that prescribing an apple a day to all adults aged fifty and over would prevent or delay around 8500 vascular deaths such as heart attacks and strokes each and every year in a country the size of England.

Apples contain vitamin C. Vitamin C is great for your immune system too. Some people lacking vitamin C in their diet have poor healing, bruise easily, and have bleeding gums. Imagine that apples also act as a toothbrush and mouthwash, thus cleaning the teeth and killing most bacteria in the mouth.

Do you have bleeding gums? The juice in an apple has properties that war against bacteria in the mouth and gums. It helps prevent tooth decay. Did I hear you ask for an apple?

Apples are low in calories. Foods that are low in calorie density are some of the trademarks of health. This is because when a food is low in calorie density we tend to eat good-sized portions and still ingest relatively few calories.

Apples are rich in boron. This nutrient is found in abundance in apples. Boron supports strong bones and a healthy and better-functioning brain. It protects your brain from brain diseases. This is something many people don't know, and when you consider that your brain makes you the person you are, it gives a whole new perspective. Apple are packed with substances called phytonutrients, and these helps to prevent neurodegenerative diseases like Alzheimer's and Parkinson's. Eat an apple a day.

Apples help prevent various cancers. Apples help in the prevention of multiple cancers like colon cancer, prostate cancer, and breast cancer in women.

Apples help the lungs. Research at the University of Nottingham shows that people who eat five or more per apples a week have fewer respiratory problems, including asthma.

Apples taste great. You could turn them into snacks. Try a slice dipped in peanut butter. They taste great. By the way, apples come in many flavors and colors:

green, yellow, or red. The taste varies greatly, but an apple is an apple that provides you with all the apple benefits--after all, variety is an important element to *maintaining good health.*

On average, Americans consume around twenty pounds of apples a year, which comes to around one apple a week. Unfortunately, while an apple a week is better than nothing, it is nowhere close to being able to extract all the advantages apples have to offer. Eating apples is part of balanced and healthy diet that would increase your longevity, so why limit yourself to only one per week? Just eat an apple a day until it becomes part of your every meal, or one meal a day.

Having said all that about an apple a day reducing the risk of diabetes, high blood pressure, and many types of cancer, would man be able to avoid the doctor entirely just by eating a bunch of this special fruit? This not likely. We might be thinking that Adam had no doctor.

If you thought so, you were mistaken. Adam and most of our progenitors had the best doctor's advice. Do not forget that God as a surgeon sliced off a rib and Eve came along. So, Adam and Eve had the best medical and natural medicine there was.

Though most studies show health benefits when we eat an apple between four and seven times a week, all our ailments cannot be cured by diet alone. In other words, we cannot elongate our lifespans like our initial forefathers. There is something else. There must be something else.

That something else is senescence--the ability of the cells to age so slowly that you don't notice it. Who knows-- Adam may not have aged at all until his DNA was modified.

What healthy changes can you make today if you are pre-diabetic or struggling with your weight?

1. Choose good foods. Eat foods that feature more vegetables and whole grains. Simply go greener. It is never a bad idea to

read nutrition facts labels.
Always search for the total
fat, saturated fat, sugar, and
sodium contents. The idea
is the lower these numbers,
the better. Buy fat-free milk
rather than regular milk.

2. You do yourself a big favor
if you leave a space for
"intelligence" in your
tummy, so to speak--if you
do not stuff yourself "fool"
of food. How much you eat,
and just not what you eat, is
very important. Small
portions help control your
weight. Even if one is
overweight, a little loss of
weight helps lower your
diabetes risk for young and
old.

3. Walk. Get moving. No
time? No problem. If you

work in a city like New York, get off the subway five or six blocks and walk fast for thirty minutes to your office. If you drive to work, park your car a thirty-minute walk away from your work location. It is the Maasai method. Exercise helps you reach and maintain good weight. You don't even have to buy expensive equipment or join a gym.

4. Do you smoke? Do you feel sad all day long? How well do you sleep? Ask your doctor for help. There are issues we cannot see that affect our diabetes risk-- things like high blood pressure, our cholesterol, and triglycerides. There are

numbers you need to know. Ask your doctor or simply research it. It is for your wellbeing.

5. Finally, ask or figure out your BMI. Are you underweight (less than 18.5), or normal weight of 18.5 to 24.9, or overweight with 25 to 29.9, or obese at 30 or greater? The earlier you know, the healthier and more forward-looking you may be.

Lengthening the human lifespan is a question of "if," not "when." The bigger question should be

"Would the gods allow man to extend his lifespan?"

Some recipes are available in Part 2 and 3 follow ups to this book.

Bibliography

Sampson, MJ. et al. Monocyte Telomere Shortening and Oxidative DNA Damage in Type 2 Diabetes. *Diabetes Care* February 2006 vol. 29 no. 2 283-289.

Adaikalakoteswari, A. et al. Association of telomere shortening with impaired glucose tolerance and diabetic macroangiopathy. *Atherosclerosis.* Vol. 195, Issue 1, Nov 2007, Pages 83-89.

Here is the link to **Hydra: Immortal** (a study by **Dr. Daniel Martinez**) *also be sure to*

explore the link provided in this dissertation for more information.
http://www.imminst.org/for um/index.php?s=&act=ST &f=48&t=884&#entry6815

A Biography on **Dr. Caleb Finch:**
http://www.usc.edu/project s/nexus/faculty/dept- ldsg/finchcaleb/finc.shtml

Research Project by **John C. Guerin- on Centenarian Species and Rock fish**.
http://www.agelessanimals. org/

Cheating Death: The Immortal Life Cycle of Turritopsis

http://www.devbio.com/article.php?ch=2&id=6